WELCOME

This Food Diary is compatible with Slimming World Plan: in your quest to lose weight and get fitter. We are positi of your day, and the helpful organised pages will keep you on track, focused and in control.

FOOD DIARY PAGE

This Food Diary has been designed to match your plan and any food variations.
Optional: Simply use the blank column headers at the top of each page for match your current plan choice. For example: Free Food, Healthy, Speed and so on.

For more detailed plan set ups - visit our website: www.myfooddiary.co.uk 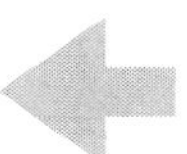

Free Food	Healthy	Speed	☕	EXTRA'S
BREAKFAST				(A)
				(B)
LUNCH				

"Blank headers will allow you to Swap Plan Formats at any time if you need to make a change or take a dieting break".

CONTENTS - EXTRA PAGES

- About You
- Weekly Weigh In
- Weight Tracking Graph
- Countdown & Mood Tracker
- Keep Busy - Get it done
- Keep Active
- Food Items and Values
- Activity Tracker - 10,000 Steps

* Online Exercise Programme

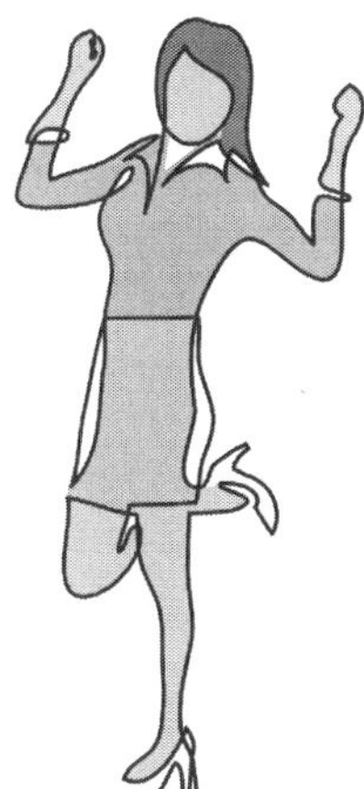

Author: Johnny Bowers / Johnny Said So

ABOUT ME

ABOUT ME: *Write down the things I like, what makes me, me?*

MY GOALS: *What are my goals... What motivates me?*

WHY: *Write down why I want to make changes in my life.*

RELAX: *What can I do to relax and unwind?*

PLAN & TREAT: *Have something to look forward to - My plans are?*

HELP: *Who can I talk to, who is going to support and help me?*

FOCUS: *Statement to myself to keep me motivated and focused!*

WEEKLY WEIGHT IN - Weeks 1 - 8

**Happy With This Weeks Results? "Tick Your Scales"*	Weight:
WEEK 1 - Date:	
"Did You Have A Good Result ?"	
WEEK 2 - Date:	
"Did You Have A Good Result ?"	
WEEK 3 - Date:	
"Did You Have A Good Result ?"	
WEEK 4 - Date:	
"Did You Have A Good Result ?"	
WEEK 5 - Date:	
"Did You Have A Good Result ?"	
WEEK 6 - Date:	
"Did You Have A Good Result ?"	
WEEK 7 - Date:	
"Did You Have A Good Result ?"	
WEEK 8 - Date:	
"Did You Have A Good Result ?"	

WEEKLY WEIGHT IN - Weeks 9 - 13

**Happy With This Weeks Results? "Tick Your Scales"*		*Weight:*
WEEK 9 - Date:		
"Did You Have A Good Result ?"		
WEEK 10 - Date:		
"Did You Have A Good Result ?"		
WEEK 11 - Date:		
"Did You Have A Good Result ?"		
WEEK 12 - Date:		
"Did You Have A Good Result ?"		
WEEK 13 - Date:		
"Did You Have A Good Result ?"		

NOTES

WEEKLY WEIGHT IN - Weeks 14 - 21

**Happy With This Weeks Results? "Tick Your Scales"*	*Weight:*
WEEK 14 - Date:	
"Did You Have A Good Result ?"	
WEEK 15 - Date:	
"Did You Have A Good Result ?"	
WEEK 16 - Date:	
"Did You Have A Good Result ?"	
WEEK 17 - Date:	
"Did You Have A Good Result ?"	
WEEK 18 - Date:	
"Did You Have A Good Result ?"	
WEEK 19 - Date:	
"Did You Have A Good Result ?"	
WEEK 20 - Date:	
"Did You Have A Good Result ?"	
WEEK 21 - Date:	
"Did You Have A Good Result ?"	

WEEKLY WEIGHT IN - Weeks 22 - 26

**Happy With This Weeks Results? "Tick Your Scales"*	Weight:
WEEK 22 - Date:	
"Did You Have A Good Result ?"	
WEEK 23 - Date:	
"Did You Have A Good Result ?"	
WEEK 24 - Date:	
"Did You Have A Good Result ?"	
WEEK 25 - Date:	
"Did You Have A Good Result ?"	
WEEK 26 - Date:	
"Did You Have A Good Result ?"	

NOTES

WEIGHT TRACKING GRAPH

Enter your "**Stone**" Weight only in **Box A** - then mark on the graph your "**Pound**" Weight!

Box A

How Much and How Fast?

You are looking to lose a healthy one to one and a half pound per week. Any more than this and your body may go into starvation mode. You want to avoid this at all costs because this may result in failure, or your weight coming back super fast as soon as your diet cycle ends. For more information about how to avoid this situation please visit: www.myfooddiary.co.uk > Select **More** from the main menu.

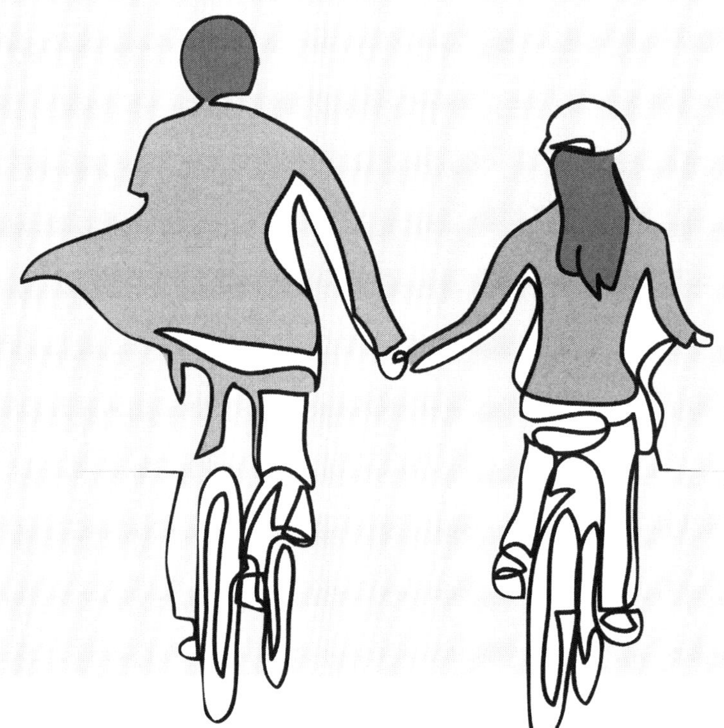

Pound Weight Marker

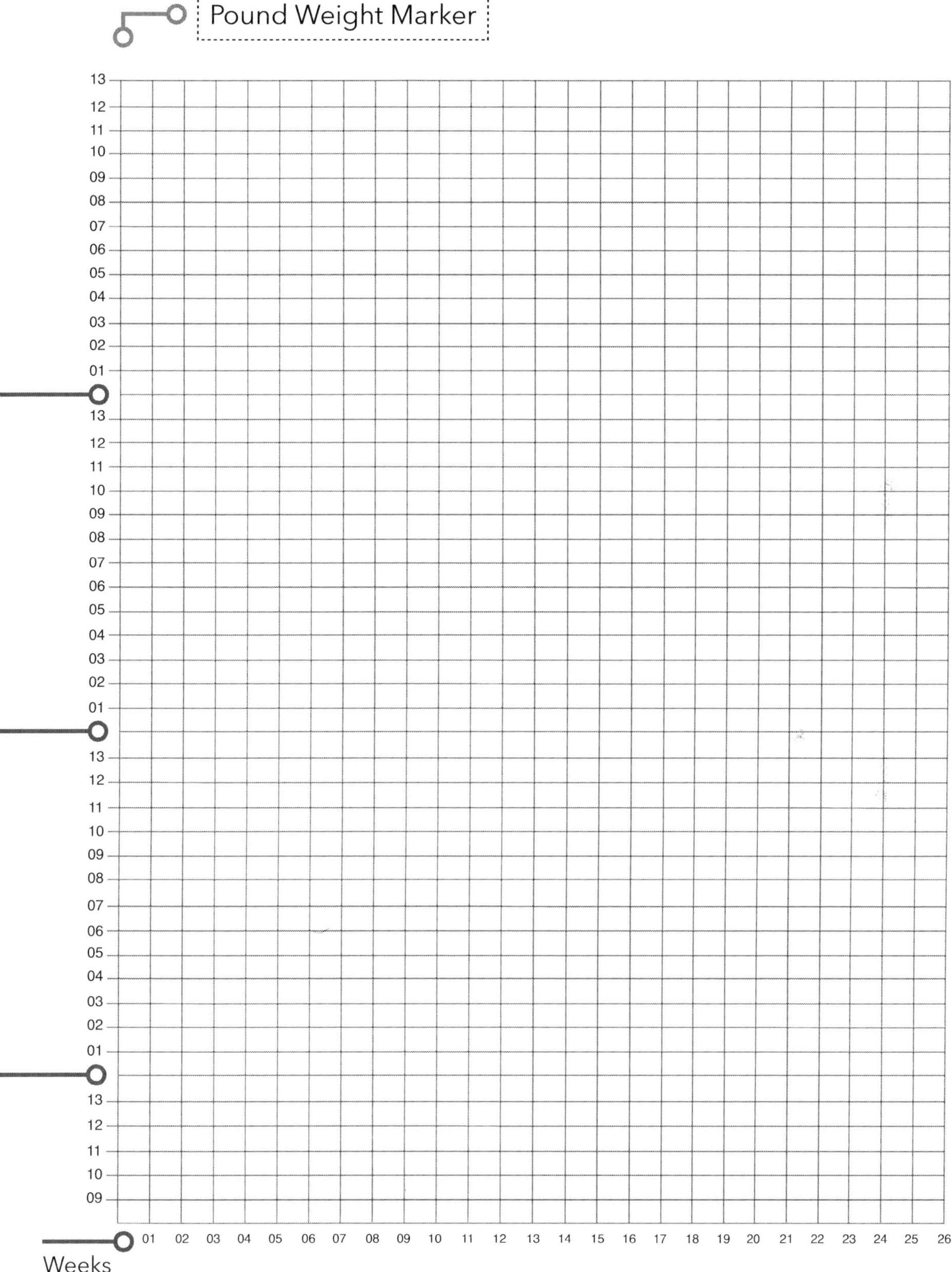

COUNTDOWN & MOOD TRACKER

26 Weeks Line a Smile or Don't!

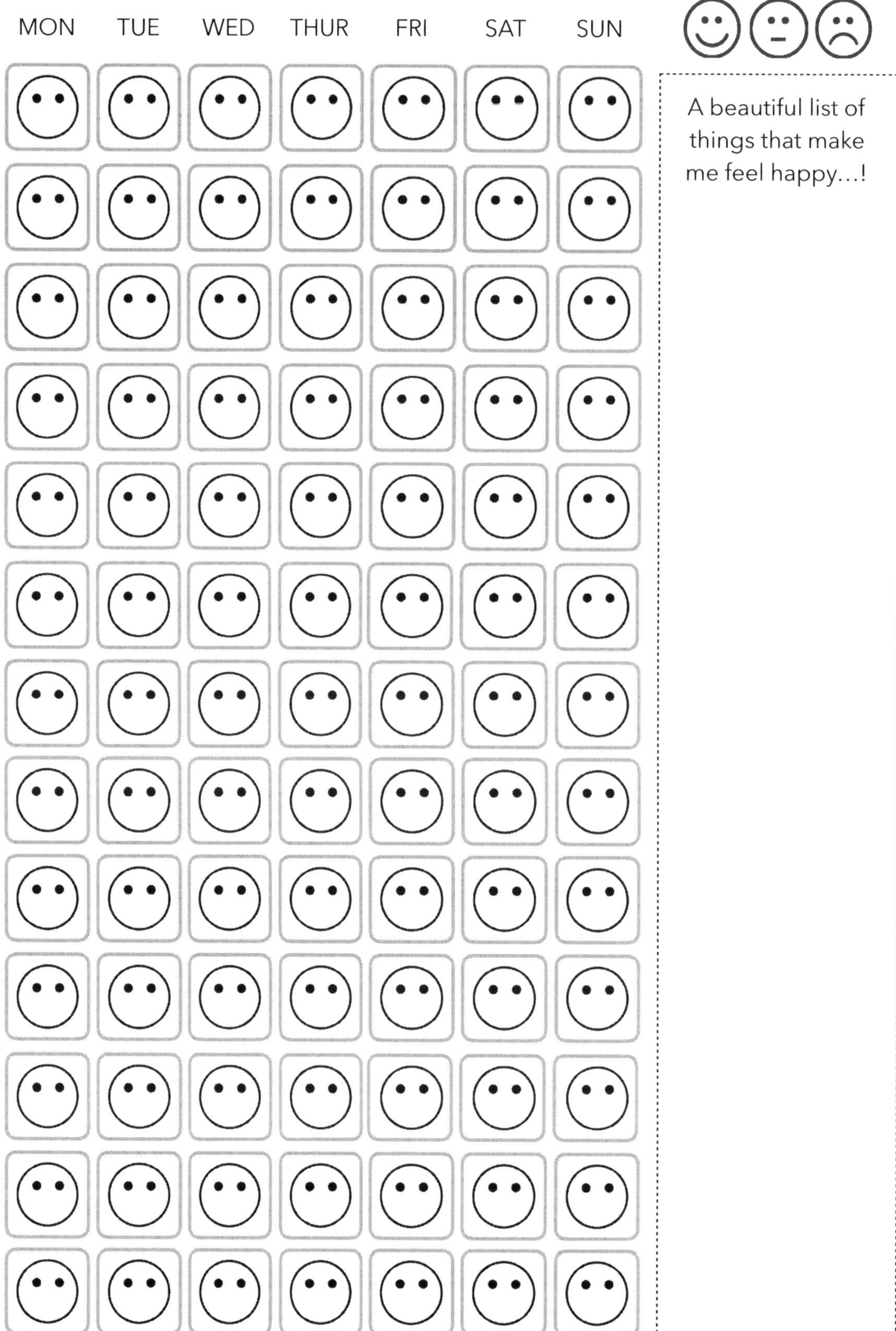

MON TUE WED THUR FRI SAT SUN

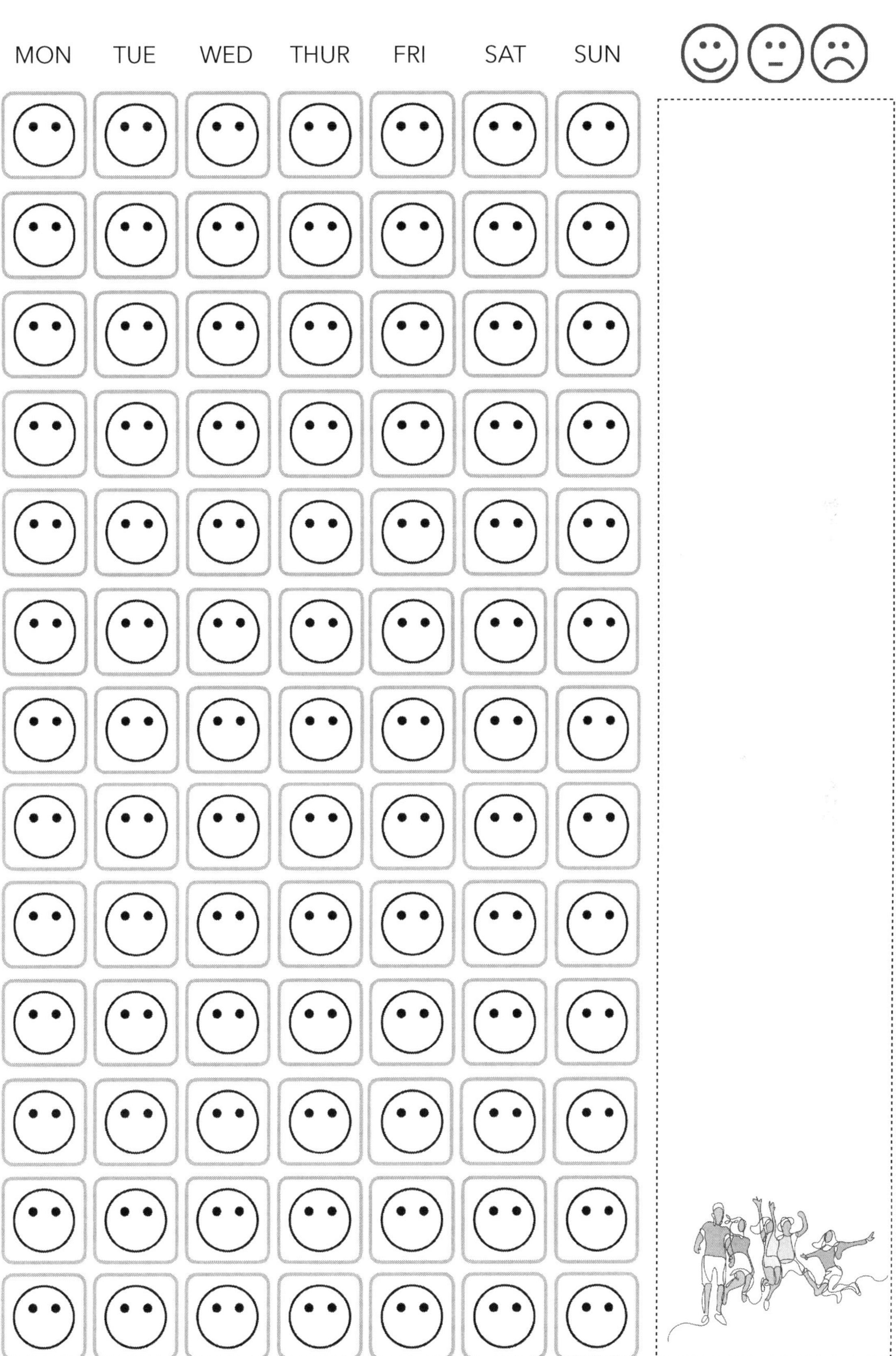

GET IT DONE...! Active Body & Mind - Jobs that will keep me busy!

- [ ]
- [ ]
- [ ]
- [ ]
- [ ]
- [ ]
- [ ]
- [ ]
- [ ]
- [ ]
- [ ]
- [ ]
- [ ]

NOTES

Activities that will help keep me busy!

NOTES

FOOD VALUE REMINDERS

Write down your most used food items and the (**SY**) values.

ITEM	VALUE	ITEM	VALUE

ITEM	VALUE

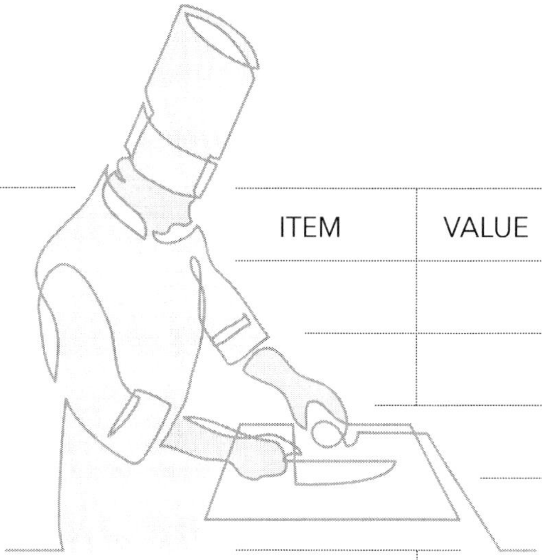

ITEM	VALUE

EXTRA'S

BREAKFAST

(A)

(B)

LUNCH

(SY) - VALUE

DINNER

Visit our website for information about "Beverage Tracking"

TOTAL

EXTRA'S

BREAKFAST

(A)

(B)

LUNCH

(SY) - VALUE

DINNER

TOTAL

EXTRA'S

BREAKFAST

(A)

(B)

LUNCH

(SY) - VALUE

DINNER

TOTAL

EXTRA'S

BREAKFAST

(A)

(B)

LUNCH

(SY) - VALUE

DINNER

TOTAL

EXTRA'S

BREAKFAST

(A)

(B)

LUNCH

(SY) - VALUE

DINNER

TOTAL

EXTRA'S

BREAKFAST

(A)

(B)

LUNCH

(SY) - VALUE

DINNER

TOTAL

EXTRA'S

BREAKFAST

(A)

(B)

LUNCH

(SY) - VALUE

DINNER

TOTAL

EXTRA'S

BREAKFAST

(A)

(B)

LUNCH

(SY) - VALUE

DINNER

TOTAL

EXTRA'S

BREAKFAST

(A)

(B)

LUNCH

(SY) - VALUE

DINNER

TOTAL

EXTRA'S

BREAKFAST

(A)

(B)

LUNCH

(SY) - VALUE

DINNER

TOTAL

EXTRA'S

BREAKFAST

(A)

(B)

LUNCH

(SY) - VALUE

DINNER

TOTAL

EXTRA'S

BREAKFAST

(A)

(B)

LUNCH

(SY) - VALUE

DINNER

TOTAL

EXTRA'S

BREAKFAST

(A)

(B)

LUNCH

(SY) - VALUE

DINNER

TOTAL

EXTRA'S

BREAKFAST

(A)

(B)

LUNCH

(SY) - VALUE

DINNER

TOTAL

EXTRA'S

BREAKFAST

(A)

(B)

LUNCH

(SY) - VALUE

DINNER

TOTAL

EXTRA'S

BREAKFAST

(A)

(B)

LUNCH

(SY) - VALUE

DINNER

TOTAL

EXTRA'S

BREAKFAST

(A)

(B)

LUNCH

(SY) - VALUE

DINNER

TOTAL

EXTRA'S

BREAKFAST

(A)

(B)

LUNCH

(SY) - VALUE

DINNER

TOTAL

EXTRA'S

BREAKFAST

(A)

(B)

LUNCH

(SY) - VALUE

DINNER

TOTAL

EXTRA'S

BREAKFAST

(A)

(B)

LUNCH

(SY) - VALUE

DINNER

TOTAL

EXTRA'S

BREAKFAST

(A)

(B)

LUNCH

(SY) - VALUE

DINNER

TOTAL

EXTRA'S

BREAKFAST

(A)

(B)

LUNCH

(SY) - VALUE

DINNER

TOTAL

EXTRA'S

BREAKFAST

(A)

(B)

LUNCH

(SY) - VALUE

DINNER

TOTAL

EXTRA'S

BREAKFAST

(A)

(B)

LUNCH

(SY) - VALUE

DINNER

TOTAL

EXTRA'S

BREAKFAST

(A)

(B)

LUNCH

(SY) - VALUE

DINNER

TOTAL

EXTRA'S

BREAKFAST

(A)

(B)

LUNCH

(SY) - VALUE

DINNER

TOTAL

EXTRA'S

BREAKFAST

(A)

(B)

LUNCH

(SY) - VALUE

DINNER

TOTAL

EXTRA'S

BREAKFAST

(A)

(B)

LUNCH

(SY) - VALUE

DINNER

TOTAL

EXTRA'S

BREAKFAST

(A)

(B)

LUNCH

(SY) - VALUE

DINNER

TOTAL

EXTRA'S

BREAKFAST

(A)

(B)

LUNCH

(SY) - VALUE

DINNER

TOTAL

EXTRA'S

BREAKFAST

(A)

(B)

LUNCH

(SY) - VALUE

DINNER

TOTAL

EXTRA'S

BREAKFAST

(A)

(B)

LUNCH

(SY) - VALUE

DINNER

TOTAL

EXTRA'S

BREAKFAST

(A)

(B)

LUNCH

(SY) - VALUE

DINNER

TOTAL

EXTRA'S

BREAKFAST

(A)

(B)

LUNCH

(SY) - VALUE

DINNER

TOTAL

EXTRA'S

BREAKFAST

(A)

(B)

LUNCH

(SY) - VALUE

DINNER

TOTAL

EXTRA'S

BREAKFAST

(A)

(B)

LUNCH

(SY) - VALUE

DINNER

TOTAL

EXTRA'S

BREAKFAST

(A)

(B)

LUNCH

(SY) - VALUE

DINNER

TOTAL

EXTRA'S

BREAKFAST

(A)

(B)

LUNCH

(SY) - VALUE

DINNER

TOTAL

EXTRA'S

BREAKFAST

(A)

(B)

LUNCH

(SY) - VALUE

DINNER

TOTAL

EXTRA'S

BREAKFAST

(A)

(B)

LUNCH

(SY) - VALUE

DINNER

TOTAL

EXTRA'S

BREAKFAST

(A)

(B)

LUNCH

(SY) - VALUE

DINNER

TOTAL

EXTRA'S

BREAKFAST

(A)

(B)

LUNCH

(SY) - VALUE

DINNER

TOTAL

EXTRA'S

BREAKFAST

(A)

(B)

LUNCH

(SY) - VALUE

DINNER

TOTAL

EXTRA'S

BREAKFAST

(A)

(B)

LUNCH

(SY) - VALUE

DINNER

TOTAL

EXTRA'S

BREAKFAST

(A)

(B)

LUNCH

(SY) - VALUE

DINNER

TOTAL

EXTRA'S

BREAKFAST

(A)

(B)

LUNCH

(SY) - VALUE

DINNER

TOTAL

EXTRA'S

BREAKFAST

(A)

(B)

LUNCH

(SY) - VALUE

DINNER

TOTAL

EXTRA'S

BREAKFAST

(A)

(B)

LUNCH

(SY) - VALUE

DINNER

TOTAL

EXTRA'S

BREAKFAST

(A)

(B)

LUNCH

(SY) - VALUE

DINNER

TOTAL

EXTRA'S

BREAKFAST

(A)

(B)

LUNCH

(SY) - VALUE

DINNER

TOTAL

EXTRA'S

BREAKFAST

(A)

(B)

LUNCH

(SY) - VALUE

DINNER

TOTAL

EXTRA'S

BREAKFAST

(A)

(B)

LUNCH

(SY) - VALUE

DINNER

TOTAL

EXTRA'S

BREAKFAST

(A)

(B)

LUNCH

(SY) - VALUE

DINNER

TOTAL

EXTRA'S

BREAKFAST

(A)

(B)

LUNCH

(SY) - VALUE

DINNER

TOTAL

EXTRA'S

BREAKFAST

(A)

(B)

LUNCH

(SY) - VALUE

DINNER

TOTAL

EXTRA'S

BREAKFAST

(A)

(B)

LUNCH

(SY) - VALUE

DINNER

TOTAL

EXTRA'S

BREAKFAST

(A)

(B)

LUNCH

(SY) - VALUE

DINNER

TOTAL

EXTRA'S

BREAKFAST

(A)

(B)

LUNCH

(SY) - VALUE

DINNER

TOTAL

EXTRA'S

BREAKFAST

(A)

(B)

LUNCH

(SY) - VALUE

DINNER

TOTAL

EXTRA'S

BREAKFAST

(A)

(B)

LUNCH

(SY) - VALUE

DINNER

TOTAL

EXTRA'S

BREAKFAST

(A)

(B)

LUNCH

(SY) - VALUE

DINNER

TOTAL

EXTRA'S

BREAKFAST

(A)

(B)

LUNCH

(SY) - VALUE

DINNER

TOTAL

EXTRA'S

BREAKFAST

(A)

(B)

LUNCH

(SY) - VALUE

DINNER

TOTAL

EXTRA'S

BREAKFAST

(A)

(B)

LUNCH

(SY) - VALUE

DINNER

TOTAL

EXTRA'S

BREAKFAST

(A)

(B)

LUNCH

(SY) - VALUE

DINNER

TOTAL

EXTRA'S

BREAKFAST

(A)

(B)

LUNCH

(SY) - VALUE

DINNER

TOTAL

EXTRA'S

BREAKFAST

(A)

(B)

LUNCH

(SY) - VALUE

DINNER

TOTAL

EXTRA'S

BREAKFAST

(A)

(B)

LUNCH

(SY) - VALUE

DINNER

TOTAL

EXTRA'S

BREAKFAST

(A)

(B)

LUNCH

(SY) - VALUE

DINNER

TOTAL

EXTRA'S

BREAKFAST

(A)

(B)

LUNCH

(SY) - VALUE

DINNER

TOTAL

EXTRA'S

BREAKFAST

(A)

(B)

LUNCH

(SY) - VALUE

DINNER

TOTAL

EXTRA'S

BREAKFAST

(A)

(B)

LUNCH

(SY) - VALUE

DINNER

TOTAL

EXTRA'S

BREAKFAST

(A)

(B)

LUNCH

(SY) - VALUE

DINNER

TOTAL

EXTRA'S

BREAKFAST

(A)

(B)

LUNCH

(SY) - VALUE

DINNER

TOTAL

EXTRA'S

BREAKFAST

(A)

(B)

LUNCH

(SY) - VALUE

DINNER

TOTAL

EXTRA'S

BREAKFAST

(A)

(B)

LUNCH

(SY) - VALUE

DINNER

TOTAL

EXTRA'S

BREAKFAST

(A)

(B)

LUNCH

(SY) - VALUE

DINNER

TOTAL

EXTRA'S

BREAKFAST

(A)

(B)

LUNCH

(SY) - VALUE

DINNER

TOTAL

EXTRA'S

BREAKFAST

(A)

(B)

LUNCH

(SY) - VALUE

DINNER

TOTAL

EXTRA'S

BREAKFAST

(A)

(B)

LUNCH

(SY) - VALUE

DINNER

TOTAL

EXTRA'S

BREAKFAST

(A)

(B)

LUNCH

(SY) - VALUE

DINNER

TOTAL

EXTRA'S

BREAKFAST

(A)

(B)

LUNCH

(SY) - VALUE

DINNER

TOTAL

EXTRA'S

BREAKFAST

(A)

(B)

LUNCH

(SY) - VALUE

DINNER

TOTAL

EXTRA'S

BREAKFAST

(A)

(B)

LUNCH

(SY) - VALUE

DINNER

TOTAL

EXTRA'S

BREAKFAST

(A)

(B)

LUNCH

(SY) - VALUE

DINNER

TOTAL

EXTRA'S

BREAKFAST

(A)

(B)

LUNCH

(SY) - VALUE

DINNER

TOTAL

EXTRA'S

BREAKFAST

(A)

(B)

LUNCH

(SY) - VALUE

DINNER

TOTAL

EXTRA'S

BREAKFAST

(A)

(B)

LUNCH

(SY) - VALUE

DINNER

TOTAL

EXTRA'S

BREAKFAST

(A)

(B)

LUNCH

(SY) - VALUE

DINNER

TOTAL

EXTRA'S

BREAKFAST

(A)

(B)

LUNCH

(SY) - VALUE

DINNER

TOTAL

EXTRA'S

BREAKFAST

(A)

(B)

LUNCH

(SY) - VALUE

DINNER

TOTAL

EXTRA'S

BREAKFAST

(A)

(B)

LUNCH

(SY) - VALUE

DINNER

TOTAL

EXTRA'S

BREAKFAST

(A)

(B)

LUNCH

(SY) - VALUE

DINNER

TOTAL

EXTRA'S

BREAKFAST

(A)

(B)

LUNCH

(SY) - VALUE

DINNER

TOTAL

EXTRA'S

BREAKFAST

(A)

(B)

LUNCH

(SY) - VALUE

DINNER

TOTAL

EXTRA'S

BREAKFAST

(A)

(B)

LUNCH

(SY) - VALUE

DINNER

TOTAL

BREAKFAST

LUNCH

DINNER

EXTRA'S

(A)

(B)

(SY) - VALUE

TOTAL

BREAKFAST

LUNCH

DINNER

EXTRA'S

(A)

(B)

(SY) - VALUE

TOTAL

EXTRA'S

BREAKFAST

(A)

(B)

LUNCH

(SY) - VALUE

DINNER

TOTAL

EXTRA'S

BREAKFAST

(A)

(B)

LUNCH

(SY) - VALUE

DINNER

TOTAL

EXTRA'S

BREAKFAST

(A)

(B)

LUNCH

(SY) - VALUE

DINNER

TOTAL

EXTRA'S

BREAKFAST

(A)

(B)

LUNCH

(SY) - VALUE

DINNER

TOTAL

EXTRA'S

BREAKFAST

(A)

(B)

LUNCH

(SY) - VALUE

DINNER

TOTAL

EXTRA'S

BREAKFAST

(A)

(B)

LUNCH

(SY) - VALUE

DINNER

TOTAL

EXTRA'S

BREAKFAST

(A)

(B)

LUNCH

(SY) - VALUE

DINNER

TOTAL

EXTRA'S

BREAKFAST

(A)

(B)

LUNCH

(SY) - VALUE

DINNER

TOTAL

EXTRA'S

BREAKFAST

(A)

(B)

LUNCH

(SY) - VALUE

DINNER

TOTAL

EXTRA'S

BREAKFAST

(A)

(B)

LUNCH

(SY) - VALUE

DINNER

TOTAL

EXTRA'S

BREAKFAST

(A)

(B)

LUNCH

(SY) - VALUE

DINNER

TOTAL

EXTRA'S

BREAKFAST

(A)

(B)

LUNCH

(SY) - VALUE

DINNER

TOTAL

EXTRA'S

BREAKFAST

(A)

(B)

LUNCH

(SY) - VALUE

DINNER

TOTAL

EXTRA'S

BREAKFAST

(A)

(B)

LUNCH

(SY) - VALUE

DINNER

TOTAL

EXTRA'S

BREAKFAST

(A)

(B)

LUNCH

(SY) - VALUE

DINNER

TOTAL

EXTRA'S

BREAKFAST

(A)

(B)

LUNCH

(SY) - VALUE

DINNER

TOTAL

EXTRA'S

BREAKFAST

(A)

(B)

LUNCH

(SY) - VALUE

DINNER

TOTAL

EXTRA'S

BREAKFAST

(A)

(B)

LUNCH

(SY) - VALUE

DINNER

TOTAL

BREAKFAST

LUNCH

DINNER

EXTRA'S

(A)

(B)

(SY) - VALUE

TOTAL

BREAKFAST

LUNCH

DINNER

EXTRA'S

(A)

(B)

(SY) - VALUE

TOTAL

EXTRA'S

BREAKFAST

(A)

(B)

LUNCH

(SY) - VALUE

DINNER

TOTAL

EXTRA'S

BREAKFAST

(A)

(B)

LUNCH

(SY) - VALUE

DINNER

TOTAL

EXTRA'S

BREAKFAST

(A)

(B)

LUNCH

(SY) - VALUE

DINNER

TOTAL

EXTRA'S

BREAKFAST

(A)

(B)

LUNCH

(SY) - VALUE

DINNER

TOTAL

EXTRA'S

BREAKFAST

(A)

(B)

LUNCH

(SY) - VALUE

DINNER

TOTAL

EXTRA'S

BREAKFAST

(A)

(B)

LUNCH

(SY) - VALUE

DINNER

TOTAL

EXTRA'S

BREAKFAST

(A)

(B)

LUNCH

(SY) - VALUE

DINNER

TOTAL

EXTRA'S

BREAKFAST

(A)

(B)

LUNCH

(SY) - VALUE

DINNER

TOTAL

EXTRA'S

BREAKFAST

(A)

(B)

LUNCH

(SY) - VALUE

DINNER

TOTAL

EXTRA'S

BREAKFAST

(A)

(B)

LUNCH

(SY) - VALUE

DINNER

TOTAL

EXTRA'S

BREAKFAST

(A)

(B)

LUNCH

(SY) - VALUE

DINNER

Visit our website for information about "Beverage Tracking"

TOTAL

EXTRA'S

BREAKFAST

(A)

(B)

LUNCH

(SY) - VALUE

DINNER

TOTAL

EXTRA'S

BREAKFAST

(A)

(B)

LUNCH

(SY) - VALUE

DINNER

TOTAL

EXTRA'S

BREAKFAST

(A)

(B)

LUNCH

(SY) - VALUE

DINNER

TOTAL

EXTRA'S

BREAKFAST

(A)

(B)

LUNCH

(SY) - VALUE

DINNER

TOTAL

EXTRA'S

BREAKFAST

(A)

(B)

LUNCH

(SY) - VALUE

DINNER

TOTAL

EXTRA'S

BREAKFAST

(A)

(B)

LUNCH

(SY) - VALUE

DINNER

TOTAL

EXTRA'S

BREAKFAST

(A)

(B)

LUNCH

(SY) - VALUE

DINNER

TOTAL

EXTRA'S

BREAKFAST

(A)

(B)

LUNCH

(SY) - VALUE

DINNER

TOTAL

EXTRA'S

BREAKFAST

(A)

(B)

LUNCH

(SY) - VALUE

DINNER

TOTAL

EXTRA'S

BREAKFAST

(A)

(B)

LUNCH

(SY) - VALUE

DINNER

TOTAL

EXTRA'S

BREAKFAST

(A)

(B)

LUNCH

(SY) - VALUE

DINNER

TOTAL

EXTRA'S

BREAKFAST

(A)

(B)

LUNCH

(SY) - VALUE

DINNER

TOTAL

EXTRA'S

BREAKFAST

(A)

(B)

LUNCH

(SY) - VALUE

DINNER

TOTAL

EXTRA'S

BREAKFAST

(A)

(B)

LUNCH

(SY) - VALUE

DINNER

TOTAL

EXTRA'S

BREAKFAST

(A)

(B)

LUNCH

(SY) - VALUE

DINNER

TOTAL

EXTRA'S

BREAKFAST

(A)

(B)

LUNCH

(SY) - VALUE

DINNER

TOTAL

EXTRA'S

BREAKFAST

(A)

(B)

LUNCH

(SY) - VALUE

DINNER

TOTAL

EXTRA'S

BREAKFAST

(A)

(B)

LUNCH

(SY) - VALUE

DINNER

TOTAL

EXTRA'S

BREAKFAST

(A)

(B)

LUNCH

(SY) - VALUE

DINNER

TOTAL

EXTRA'S

BREAKFAST

(A)

(B)

LUNCH

(SY) - VALUE

DINNER

TOTAL

EXTRA'S

BREAKFAST

(A)

(B)

LUNCH

(SY) - VALUE

DINNER

TOTAL

EXTRA'S

BREAKFAST

(A)

(B)

LUNCH

(SY) - VALUE

DINNER

TOTAL

EXTRA'S

BREAKFAST

(A)

(B)

LUNCH

(SY) - VALUE

DINNER

TOTAL

EXTRA'S

BREAKFAST

(A)

(B)

LUNCH

(SY) - VALUE

DINNER

TOTAL

EXTRA'S

BREAKFAST

(A)

(B)

LUNCH

(SY) - VALUE

DINNER

TOTAL

EXTRA'S

BREAKFAST

(A)

(B)

LUNCH

(SY) - VALUE

DINNER

TOTAL

EXTRA'S

BREAKFAST

(A)

(B)

LUNCH

(SY) - VALUE

DINNER

TOTAL

EXTRA'S

BREAKFAST

(A)

(B)

LUNCH

(SY) - VALUE

DINNER

TOTAL

EXTRA'S

BREAKFAST

(A)

(B)

LUNCH

(SY) - VALUE

DINNER

TOTAL

EXTRA'S

BREAKFAST

(A)

(B)

LUNCH

(SY) - VALUE

DINNER

TOTAL

EXTRA'S

BREAKFAST

(A)

(B)

LUNCH

(SY) - VALUE

DINNER

TOTAL

EXTRA'S

BREAKFAST

(A)

(B)

LUNCH

(SY) - VALUE

DINNER

TOTAL

EXTRA'S

BREAKFAST

(A)

(B)

LUNCH

(SY) - VALUE

DINNER

TOTAL

EXTRA'S

BREAKFAST

(A)

(B)

LUNCH

(SY) - VALUE

DINNER

TOTAL

EXTRA'S

BREAKFAST

(A)

(B)

LUNCH

(SY) - VALUE

DINNER

TOTAL

EXTRA'S

BREAKFAST

(A)

(B)

LUNCH

(SY) - VALUE

DINNER

TOTAL

EXTRA'S

BREAKFAST

(A)

(B)

LUNCH

(SY) - VALUE

DINNER

TOTAL

EXTRA'S

BREAKFAST

(A)

(B)

LUNCH

(SY) - VALUE

DINNER

TOTAL

EXTRA'S

BREAKFAST

(A)

(B)

LUNCH

(SY) - VALUE

DINNER

TOTAL

EXTRA'S

BREAKFAST

(A)

(B)

LUNCH

(SY) - VALUE

DINNER

TOTAL

EXTRA'S

BREAKFAST

(A)

(B)

LUNCH

(SY) - VALUE

DINNER

TOTAL

EXTRA'S

BREAKFAST

(A)

(B)

LUNCH

(SY) - VALUE

DINNER

TOTAL

EXTRA'S

BREAKFAST

(A)

(B)

LUNCH

(SY) - VALUE

DINNER

TOTAL

EXTRA'S

BREAKFAST

(A)

(B)

LUNCH

(SY) - VALUE

DINNER

TOTAL

EXTRA'S

BREAKFAST

(A)

(B)

LUNCH

(SY) - VALUE

DINNER

TOTAL

EXTRA'S

BREAKFAST

(A)

(B)

LUNCH

(SY) - VALUE

DINNER

TOTAL

EXTRA'S

BREAKFAST

(A)

(B)

LUNCH

(SY) - VALUE

DINNER

TOTAL

EXTRA'S

BREAKFAST

(A)

(B)

LUNCH

(SY) - VALUE

DINNER

TOTAL

EXTRA'S

BREAKFAST

(A)

(B)

LUNCH

(SY) - VALUE

DINNER

TOTAL

EXTRA'S

BREAKFAST

(A)

(B)

LUNCH

(SY) - VALUE

DINNER

TOTAL

EXTRA'S

BREAKFAST

(A)

(B)

LUNCH

(SY) - VALUE

DINNER

TOTAL

EXTRA'S

BREAKFAST

(A)

(B)

LUNCH

(SY) - VALUE

DINNER

TOTAL

EXTRA'S

BREAKFAST

(A)

(B)

LUNCH

(SY) - VALUE

DINNER

TOTAL

EXTRA'S

BREAKFAST

(A)

(B)

LUNCH

(SY) - VALUE

DINNER

TOTAL

EXTRA'S

BREAKFAST

(A)

(B)

LUNCH

(SY) - VALUE

DINNER

TOTAL

ACTIVITY TRACKER - 10,000 STEPS...!

So where does the magic number come from? It's believed that the concept of 10,000 steps originated in Japan in the run-up to the 1964 Tokyo Olympics, says Catrine Tudor-Locke, an associate professor at the Pennington Biomedical Research Centre at Louisiana State University.

Pedometers became all the rage in the country as Olympic fever swept through Japanese society. One company came out with a device called a manpo-kei, which means 10,000 step meter.

Since then 10,000 steps has become a commonly-acknowledged goal for daily fitness across the world. The 10,000-step goal could be just right for you – and the benefits of a 30-minute extra walk to help hit your target helps:

- Lowers blood pressure
- Lowers depression
- Improves Sleep
- And makes you Super Fit

Set your goal and build up to the 10,000 steps per day.

Our activity tracker is set up so it acts like a graph allowing you to see your daily step totals at a glance.

Steps Range - 6 to 12,000 Steps - The Centre Grey Box / Line is the Goal

For more information and to see a Graph Example: www.myfooddiary.co.uk
Select **>More** and then see **Activity Tracker**

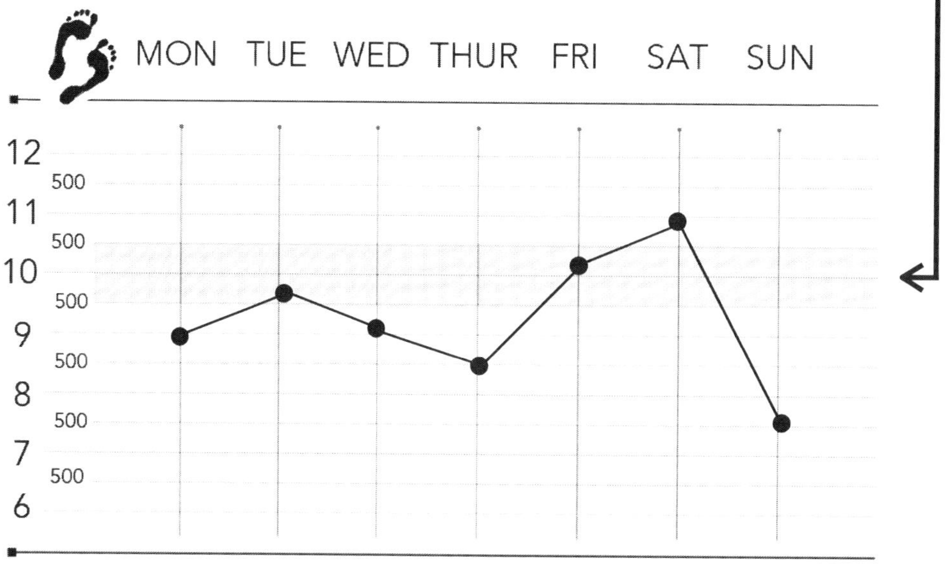

MON TUE WED THUR FRI SAT SUN

12
500
11
500
10
500
9
500
8
500
7
500
6

12
500
11
500
10
500
9
500
8
500
7
500
6

12
500
11
500
10
500
9
500
8
500
7
500
6

12
500
11
500
10
500
9
500
8
500
7
500
6

12
500
11
500
10
500
9
500
8
500
7
500
6

MON TUE WED THUR FRI SAT SUN

12
500
11
500
10
500
9
500
8
500
7
500
6

12
500
11
500
10
500
9
500
8
500
7
500
6

12
500
11
500
10
500
9
500
8
500
7
500
6

12
500
11
500
10
500
9
500
8
500
7
500
6

12
500
11
500
10
500
9
500
8
500
7
500
6

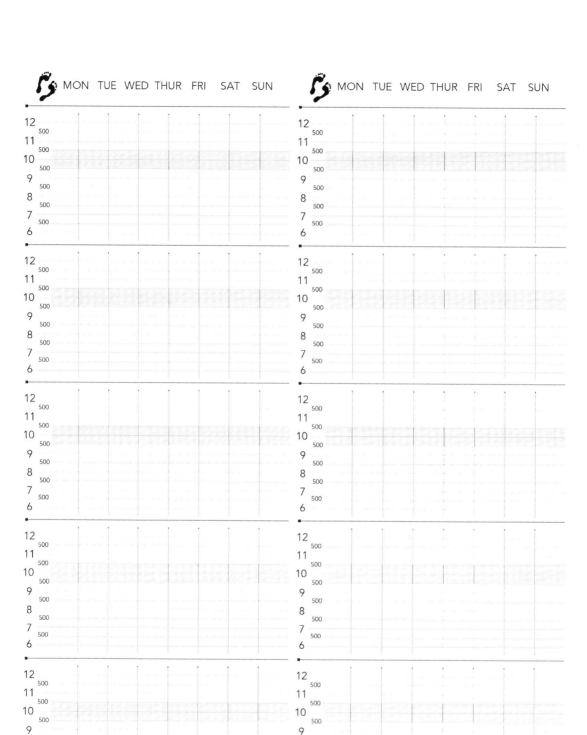

MON TUE WED THUR FRI SAT SUN

12
500
11
500
10
500
9
500
8
500
7
500
6

12
500
11
500
10
500
9
500
8
500
7
500
6

12
500
11
500
10
500
9
500
8
500
7
500
6

12
500
11
500
10
500
9
500
8
500
7
500
6

12
500
11
500
10
500
9
500
8
500
7
500
6

MON TUE WED THUR FRI SAT SUN

12
500
11
500
10
500
9
500
8
500
7
500
6

12
500
11
500
10
500
9
500
8
500
7
500
6

12
500
11
500
10
500
9
500
8
500
7
500
6

12
500
11
500
10
500
9
500
8
500
7
500
6

12
500
11
500
10
500
9
500
8
500
7
500
6

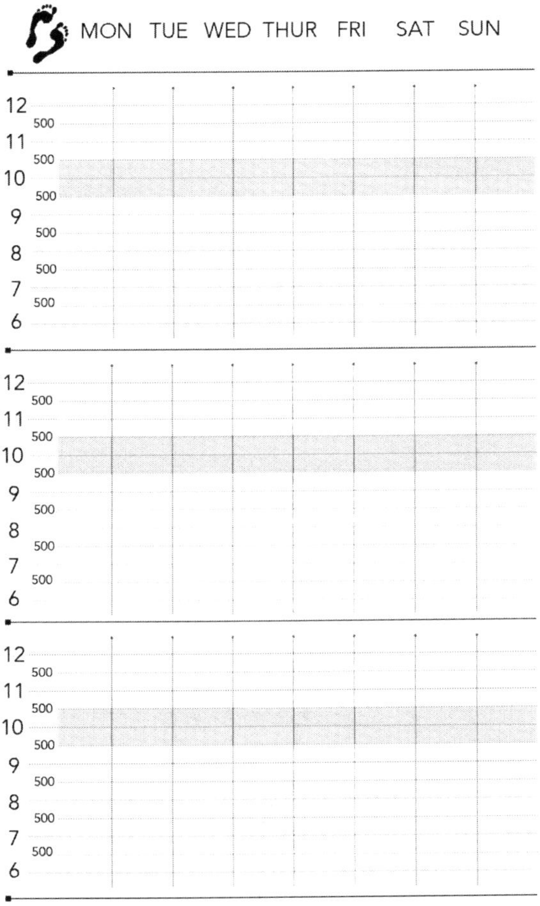

12
500
11
500
10
500
9
500
8
500
7
500
6

12
500
11
500
10
500
9
500
8
500
7
500
6

12
500
11
500
10
500
9
500
8
500
7
500
6

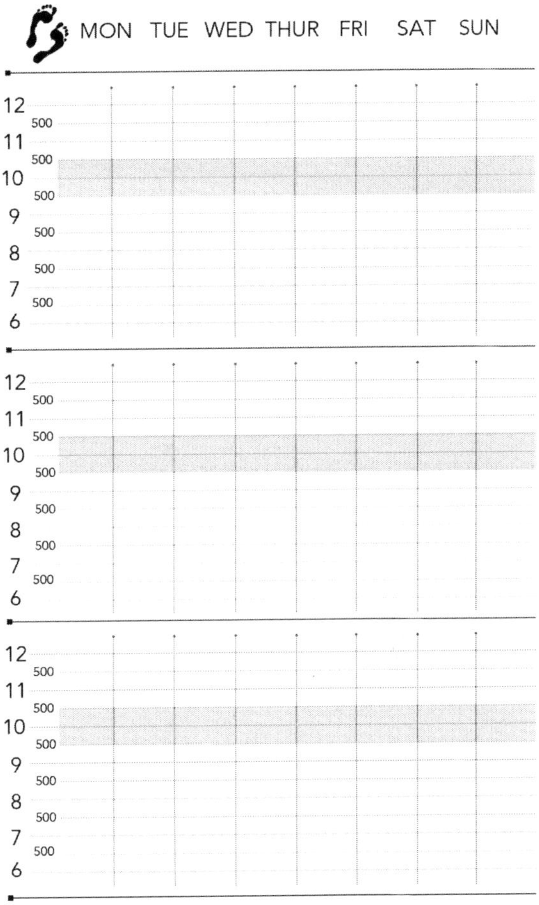

12
500
11
500
10
500
9
500
8
500
7
500
6

12
500
11
500
10
500
9
500
8
500
7
500
6

12
500
11
500
10
500
9
500
8
500
7
500
6

Printed in Great Britain
by Amazon

37331155R00063